Thanks to the r̶ ... ̶p̶e̶d̶ ̶a̶n̶d̶ will help make this book.

    First: To the Lord who I believe through my holy spirit, I was bestowed the awareness of a third energy that was the stepping stone to the structure of 3MCP.

    Next but not least to my entire family. I have editors that helped with the wording, spelling, grammar, structure and photographic imperfections.

    I have a cartoonist for a future cartoon. A professional photographer to help with a video. I am blessed with another writer that provides input.

    And to the least myself for being at the age in my life that I can enjoy the blessing that this can bring to others and it not be about myself.

Thank you Jesus.

Table of contents

Page 3:   Front Cover Photos

Page 4:   Seek and You Shall Find

Page 5-6:   My Exercise Experience

Page 7-8:   Reason behind 3MCP

Page 9:   Stepping Stones or Paths

Page 10-11:   Structure of 3MCP

Page 12:   Program Development

Page 13:   Photos of Hand Contact

Page 14:   Program Basics

Page 15:   Photos Stomach Arms and Hands

Page 16:   Stomach Routine

Page 17:   Photos Stomach Routine

Page 18:   Stomach Routine Continued

Page 19:   Photos Upper Body

Page 20:   Upper Body

Page 21:   Photos Upper Body

Page 22:   Upper Body

Page 23:   Photos Lower Body

Page 24:   Lower Body

All Rights Reserved

First Copyright © 2003 by Roger Tincher

No part of this book may be reproduced or transmitted in any form or by any means, electronic or mechanical, including photocopying, recording, or by any information storage and retrieval system without permission, in writing, from the owner Roger Tincher. Publishing and distribution rights owned in the United States of America by Roger Tincher.

Front Cover Photos

1990-2000 photo: At that time my weight was 230 lbs. I had carried that extra weight for at least ten years maybe even longer.

In the early part of 2001 I started structuring, doing, writing the program and recording results. By June of 2001 my weight was at 210 I lost 20 lbs. By the end of 2001 my weight was 200 down 10 more pounds. With the program I lost 15 pounds in 2002 and an additional 10 lbs. in 2003.

The 2003 photo: shows me at 175 lbs. the weight I graduated high school in 1968. The extended belt is showing I had reduced the circumference of my stomach by 10 inches along with excess body fat over my entire body.

The 2005 photo: shows me still at 175.

The 2013 photo: I'm at 185 lbs. a slight increase in muscle mass over the entire body.

The 2023 photo: shows me at present caring 185 to 190 lbs. depending on the time of the year.

What could have been?

The average weight gain in the United States during the holidays of October into January is 6 to10 pounds from eating the holiday treats. I am average and do like to eat. I have gained and lost over the last 23 years some 100 plus pounds not mentioned above. Meaning my weight could have been 350 to 400 plus. If I had not been using the program.

My holiday gained weight I lose by the first to the middle of March depending upon how much I gained. When I watch and control how much I eat I gain less to nothing at all.

This simple program allows one to not only experience many weight loss benefits it also provides one with control to enjoy their life as they choose. One may eat a variety of foods of their liking just watch how much.

One might enjoy their sweets if health permits just watch how often as well as how much.

This easily achievable program puts into the hands of each individual how and what they will experience and receive.

One has to get committed and that might take time. Realize that as little as one pound loss in the beginning is a positive result and a step in the right direction. The use of number counting in the program are objectives, do what is comfortable to start and strive for the objective. We are all different yet we are the same, we take in nourishment, we store some, we need to use it. Stored fat was to sustain life if needed not endanger it.

Seek and you shall find

I believe that through my Holly Spirit I was bestowed the awareness of the presence of a third energy that can be generated by the body within the body.

With the third energy and my acquired background experience. What evolved is a very simple process of losing weight and taking control of ones future health.

Three Minute Couch Potato is the composed blending of isometrics, aerobics and yoga into a gentle total body application. Three minutes at a time. It puts into the hands of any individual the opportunity to take control of their future it just takes commitment.

It is forgiving. If one gets away from it for a while all it takes is just committing again, and again, and again, however many times it takes. It can be difficult from the start and for many it will be. It may take several attempts and for many it will.

Just believe that it will if one does.

I believe that the only time it is too late, if there is no longer light in the eyes for one is no longer breathing.

Believe and commit so you too will find that I am right.

My exercise experience

My name is Roger Tincher. As of 2023 I am 73 years young and I am walking my majestic plateau. I created, developed, structured and I am the author of the low-impact full body exercise and weight loss program Three Minute Couch Potato.

I have taken the full body approach to engaging muscles all of my life. In my youth I did the typical things young boys do walked, ran, rode bikes, swam and played hard. In grade school, high school and into my 30's I participated in sports with baseball, basketball, football and softball.

At age 13 I got my first 110lb. bar bell weight set. Consisting of concrete inside plastic molds and a bar. When I started working out with the weight set I did squats, overhead presses, bench presses, curls, sit ups, just to mention a few of the multiple methods of engaging muscles over the entire body.

When working with weights you have moves that push the weight away from the body, some pull it toward the body also those that apply the pressure down through the body. There are many methods of using weights for physical muscle engagement.

My mental and physical approach to weight lifting has always been not how much I could do but how much I could control and achieve the total workout that I wanted. I started with that attitude as a teen and have maintained it through my adult life.

In high school I maintained my association with free weights as well as I started working out with dumb bells and on the universal weight machine.

Dumb bells allow single arm or double arm application with weight and increases work out options like shoulder rolls, overhead presses, isolated curls just to mention a few.

The universal machine has multiple exercise positions around the frame of the unit. This allows the user or users to work multiple body areas all on one machine. The weights on the unit for each position are located in the center area of the frame and not over the body as free weights are making it safer for the user.

After high school during trade school, college, working career and a family life I continued my full body workouts.

I replaced my old weight set with steel weights that last longer and purchased my own dumb bells. I've worked out in the gyms at school, in apartments when I lived there and joined gyms after I moved into a home.

I continued using universal machines, also incorporated individual units like stationary bikes, rowing machines, treadmills, steppers, along with other machines available. I also used free weights and dumb bells when I wanted the pressure that they produce.

In my 30's I started slowing down on my exercising at gyms not that I didn't think it was good for me it just took up so much time.

By that time I had experience working out on some form of every exercise machine and used multiple approaches to engaging muscles over the entire body.

My accumulated experience exercising over the 73 years of my life is in the thousands of hours. I do not mean for this to sound overwhelming or impressive. But I do mean it too let you the reader know that I do know what I am doing.

The reason behind 3MCP

For decades I have watched Americans and the World gaining weight. I first noticed it in the early 60's with children being teased and called names. As I got older I became aware that it was not just the teasing and the name calling but also the many health problems associated with being overweight.

This problem has no limitation. It includes all ethnic groups from children through mature adults. The grip is throughout the world and has been rapidly increasing for several decades.

Very few of the millions upon millions of men, women and children that are in the grasp of overweight to obesity want to be there. Many feel helpless with no idea of how to get control of the unhealthy problem that has captured them.

Overweight leads to multiple internal and external health issues causing many early deaths. Weight loss on the other hand has hundreds of benefits internally, externally, mentally and physically as well as financially.

There is not just one thing that has caused the overweight problem in America and the World.

To simply state the very complex makeup of the human body. Whether one believes we evolved from an ape like creature, that we came from dust in the Garden of Eden, or even that mankind just happens to be here.

To sustain life the human body must consume nourishment in the form of solids, liquids and oxygen. The internal structure than converts the ingredients into a liquid food to fuel the body. The vascular system is used to carry the liquid fuel and distribute it throughout the entire body.

The natural make up from the beginning has been to store a small amount of the fuel around muscles, internal organs, anywhere throughout the body that blood flows in the solid form of fat for survival if needed.

Over time with the discovery of fire, weapons, and salt. Food became easier to obtain, more body fuel was retained and mankind started to get heavier.

Around the industrial revolution advancements like refrigeration, ice, sitting jobs, automobiles, radio, TV, telephone for a few examples. The overweight problem started to increase at an alarming rate.

With the introduction of the transistor the world started producing computers, cell phones, microwaves, fast foods, carbonated drinks of all kinds, video games. These are but a few examples of the many things that have created more sitting jobs, time watching TV, playing video games and time behind the wheel getting to and from work. These modernizations have led to a fast paced time limiting life style that has further added to the obesity problem that has been ever increasing.

Keep in mind the body is still storing a small amount of food in the form of fat throughout the entire body.

Stepping Stones or Paths

I indicated that the grip of obesity has a grasp on million upon millions of individuals worldwide with America leading the pace.

The vast majority of the individuals finding themselves in this crisis feel helpless and lost. They want to take control of their weight issue but do not know how.

There are so many paths or stepping stones out there. But very few are for the overweight individual that initially may not have the self-confidence to reach out or the back ground knowledge to get safely started.

Diet plans do not consider the ethnic diversity that exist.

The high-impact approach to weight training has many benefits. But it also takes a lot of time away from home. In our fast pace demanding society the majority of individuals do not have the extra hours needed nor the experience to safely train.

There are several types of in-home equipment that can be purchased. They are expensive, take up a lot of room if not require their own room. Many of them end up idle, sold, or given away.

There are quick fixes like pills and surgical options. With pills a foreign chemical is added into the body and with surgery there are always risk.

There are other steps one can take like walking, swimming, riding a bike are just a few. The weather can be a restricting factor.

In the last few years' information released has shown that a low-impact workout program allows one to lose weight with minimal body fatigue, necessary for maintaining body weight loss over an extended period of time.

There has also been resent data released that just a few minutes daily of a low-impact program provides multiple health benefits.

I created this program with children in mind. I structured it to be easily achievable by individuals of all ages with no previous experience necessary.

3MCP gently engages muscles energizing them. Energized muscles absorb associated body fat for 24 to 48 hours.

Structure of 3MCP

In the early part of 90's I noticed in myself and across the country that a large percentage of the population had gotten overweight to obese. Mainly my stomach had gotten out of control along with excess body fat distributed over my entire body.

I started looking for a zero-impact way to engage muscles starting with the stomach and be able to incorporate it for the entire body. The initial requirements for the workout were that it did not stress muscles nor cause high pressure points on the joints of the body.

I initially tried two previous attempts. The first approach was in a position on the floor with the knees and upper body curled in toward each other. I induced pressure into the stomach muscles with abdominal contraction and maintaining over a period of time. This proved to be ineffective being very limited and caused too much pressure on the back. Also there was no way to progress on into the rest of the body.

My second approach was in a crawling like position on the floor with the legs bent at the knees, hands on the floor and the arms extended out in front of the body at different angles from the shoulders. This applied pressure into the abdominal muscles or stomach area but also induced an extreme amount of pressure into joints throughout the body. Making it very uncomfortable and not acceptable for long term use.

In December of 2000 from a standing position and hands clasp in front of my stomach I raised my hands up across my stomach and felt a tiny tingle of energy beneath my hands pass through the abdominal muscles.

At that moment I knew that I had found or received what I had been searching for. I do believe that the blessing was bestowed upon me by the Lord through my holy spirit.

I later realized that the searching process had progressed from a baby like position curled up on the floor, through an infant learning to crawl, and finally maturing into an upright standing position.

At that time I started developing, and structuring the workout, recording the personal progress and writing the program that would become Three Minute Couch Potato. The program gets its name from it taking 3 minutes to complete one set and couch potato being a common reference to people gaining weight while watching TV.

The requirements for the workout were that it had to be low-impact to not stress muscles, nor cause high pressure points on the joints of the body. A major requirement was that it had to be easily achievable by inexperienced overweight to obese children and individuals of all ages.

It had to be slow-paced to allow for full extension and retraction of muscles energizing them to absorb excess body fat.

3MCP does all of the above and more it relaxes sore tense muscles, extends range of motion, increases muscle definition, allows one to look and feel younger all while removing excess body fat.

These are but a few of the many benefits that one receives from weight loss.

It is performed in the safety and comfort of one's own home, does not require a lot of personal time, can be easily worked into ones daily routine. The low-impact allows it to be repeated during the day if desired. It also increases energy level making one feel better mentally and physically.

Program Development

I started looking for an easy way to engage the muscles of the body starting with the stomach. The body consists of two energy fields: the left side and the right side muscles. I discovered that by connecting the hands together, a third smaller energy was produced, and that it could be focused or channeled into the stomach muscles from a standing position. I named this 3rd energy, "the scrapping edge."

To be able to work oversized stomachs of any size, I viewed it in three vertical areas: center, left side, and right side. Each of these areas have three horizontal sections: lower, center, and upper. This way of approaching the stomach, along with a structured movement of the hands over the stomach, channels the scrapping edge produced into the muscles, energizing them.

The structure of the Three Minute Couch Potato moves the hands first over the stomach, then proceeds to the upper body, and finishes with the lower body all in a slow-paced continuous motion routine.

The slow-pace of the routine is to allow muscles to fully extend and retract. This distributes energy evenly to and through the muscles, energizing them. Energized muscles absorb surrounding body fat, while sculpting the body to its natural shape.

The low-impact design of the program provides minimal body fatigue over an extended period of time, necessary for maintaining body weight loss.

Energized muscles will reduce muscle soreness caused by stress or physical exertion, extend range of motion, and produce an increased energy level, all while losing excess body fat.

It is recommended that a doctor be consulted to see if there are any physical restrictions that need to be considered before starting a workout program.

Contact of Hands

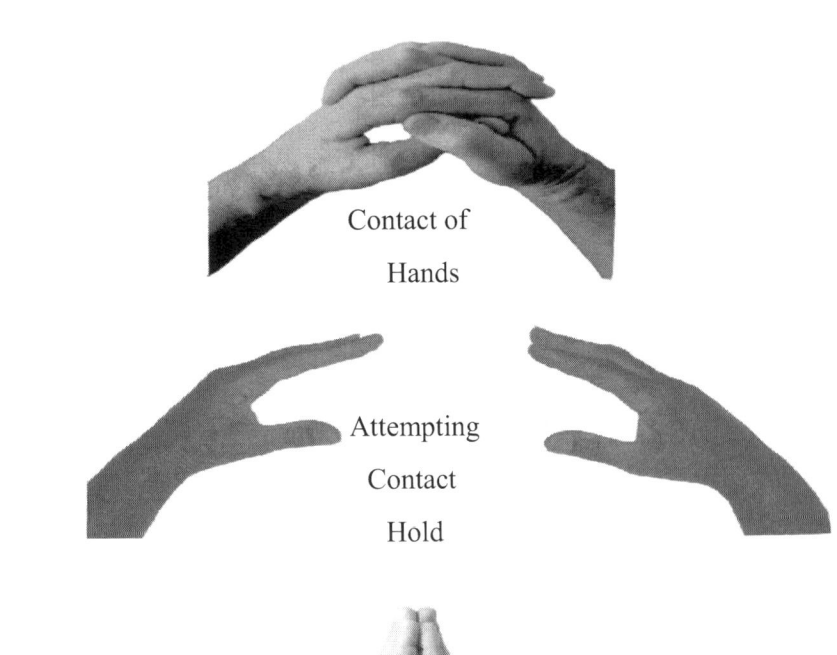

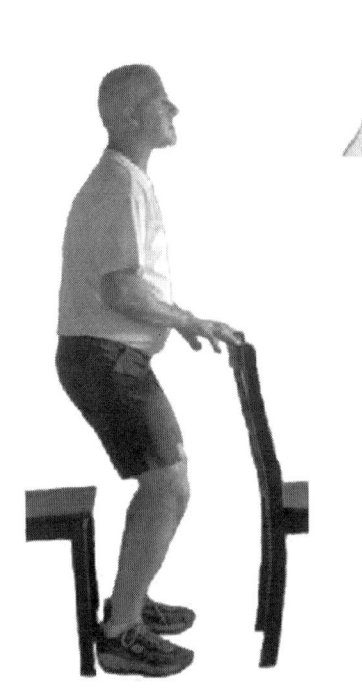

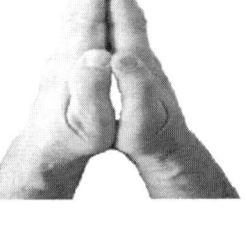

Attempting Contact Hold

Flat

Lightly touch stationary surface

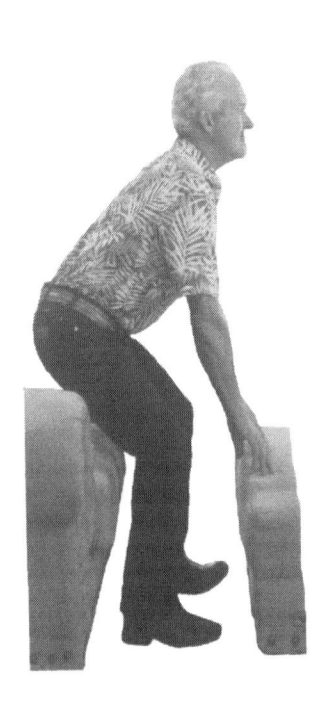

Program Basics

The programs routine is done from a comfortable standing position in front of a chair or sofa to allow for sitting down if needed. When working the lower body, a stationary object will be used to help position the upper body weight onto the legs.

While breathing through the exercise, it should be slow and even. I suggest breathing through the nose. This is to direct more air into the lungs and less air into the stomach. If it is uncomfortable to breathe through the nose, use a comfortable breathing technique.

This routine uses multiple variations of contact with the hands. One of them being the fingers of both hands touching. This approach can be anything from just touching at the finger tips to anywhere down along the sides. Using another contact, the palms and fingers of the hands are lying flat against each other with the fingers extended. In the final connection, the fingers are touching some type of stationary surface around hip height. The surface can be anything from the edge of a table to the arm or back of a chair.

If in the beginning the stomach is too large for the fingers to touch and cross, the attempting at contact and holding that position will also work. This is to be explained in more detail later.

This program energizes muscles over the entire body. It starts with the stomach, continues to the upper body, and finishes in the lower body. One set takes around three minutes from start to finish, and the program is structured to be repeated three times. Allow a little time between each set.

The program can also be combined with TV. While watching TV, when a commercial comes on you can do the routine. Three commercials and the program is completed.

This program comes with a self-imposed universal diet too complement our diverse social structure. Start first with the program and be committed, than implement the diet as needed per individual. Continue eating what one already likes to eat, limiting how much one eats and restricting when one eats. These simple steps makes a big difference with positive results.

Contact of
Hands.

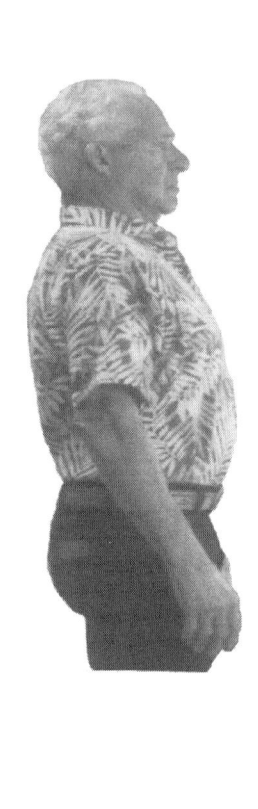

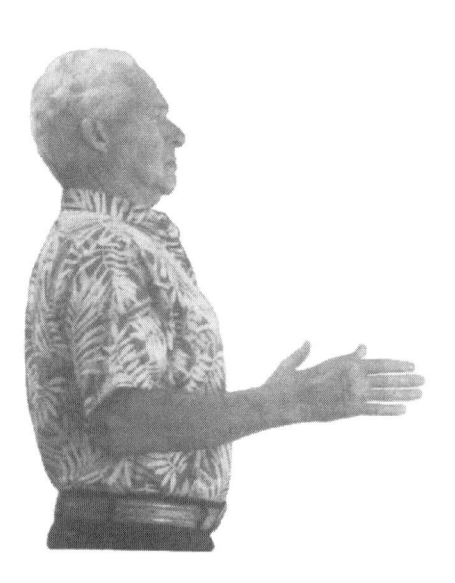

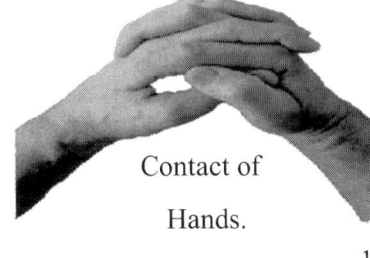

Hole attempt
to touch.

Stomach Routine

To start this program we must first start with the stomach muscles. To assist in energizing the stubborn abdominal muscles, I suggest that a slight contraction of the stomach be used during this portion of the routine. Initially the body fat surrounding these muscles makes it difficult to near impossible for individuals to feel the energy being channeled into them. The contracting of the abdominal muscles does not have to be constant. If it becomes uncomfortable, temporarily discontinue. Resume when discomfort disappears.

Start from a comfortable standing position with feet separated somewhere from hip to shoulder width apart. Do the program in front of a chair or sofa which will allow for sitting if needed. Loosely hang the arms down along each side of the body. Bend the arms at the elbow to a ninety degree angle. This will place both forearms along each side of the stomach with the hands extended out in front of the body. Rotate the hands so the palms are pointed toward each other.

Move the hands inward toward each other bringing them together in front of the stomach. Spread the fingers of both hands and cross them. The contact of the crossed fingers can be anything from just touching at the finger tips to clasping them together. This connection is meant to be loose so there is no need to grasp them tightly.

The hands need to move freely over the entire stomach. To achieve this, move the elbows out slightly from the sides of the stomach. Allow a comfortable space to exist between the inside of the arms and hands and the sides of the stomach.

If the stomach is to large at this time to cross the fingers and allow the space mentioned above, make and maintain the attempt to touch the fingers. To achieve this from the standing position, the arms should be bent at the elbows, hands extended out in front of the body. Move the hands across the front of the stomach as close as comfortably possible. Maintain the attempt to touch and cross the fingers while allowing space necessary for movement of the hands over the stomach. The attempting to cross the fingers and maintaining the attempt will energize stomach muscles.

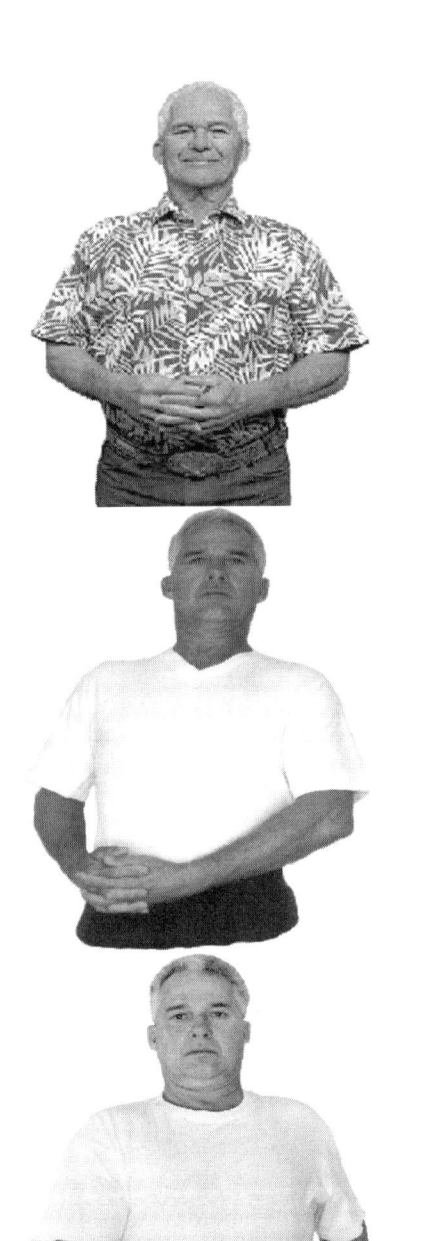

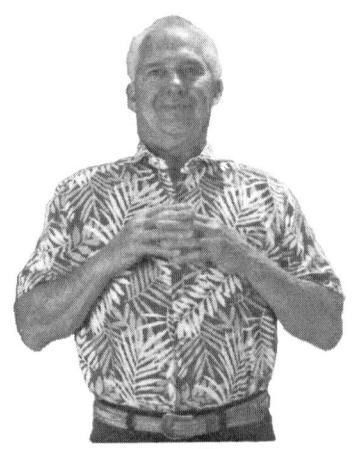

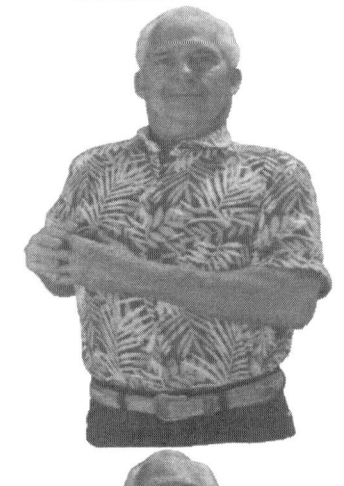

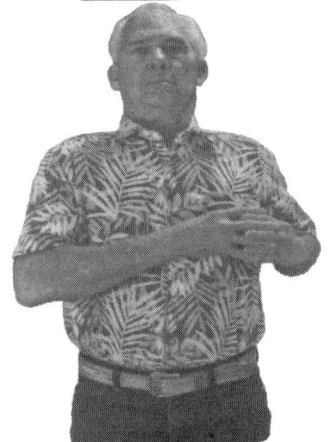

Repeat 3 times.

Repeat 3 times.

Repeat 3 times.

There is no need to force the fingers together. As the fat around the stomach muscles comes off, the hands will come closer together. At some point the fingers will touch and be able to cross.

At this time the hands are in front of the center stomach area. With the arms bent at the elbow, lower the hands below the naval into the lower section. This is the starting position for this area.

Bending the elbows, slowly raise the hands from the lower section, up across the center, to the sternum bone of the upper section and pause. Slowly lower arms back to the starting position. Repeat the upward and downward movement of the hands over the center area three times.

After completing the center area of the stomach the hands need to be moved to the right, lower starting position. This can easily be done by moving the right upper arm and elbow back, while moving the left upper arm and elbow forward. This will move the hands into the lower section of the right side. This is the starting position for this area.

Bending the elbows slowly raise the hands from the lower section, across the center, up the rib cage and pause. Slowly lower the hands back to the lower starting position for a count of one. Repeat this two more times for a total of three times.

Having worked the hands over the right side now we need to work the left. This can be done by moving the left upper arm and elbow back, while bringing forward the right upper arm and elbow moving the hands from the right side across the center into the left lower section. This is the left side starting position.

Bending the elbows, slowly raise the hands from the lower section, across the center, up the rib cage and pause. Slowly lower the hands back to the starting position for a count of one. Repeat this move two more times for a total of three times.

The hands have now gone over the stomach completely once. The program is structured for the stomach to be gone over completely three times. Move the hands back to the first used starting position of the center area and repeat moves over the center, right, and left areas two more times. Covering the entire stomach a total of three times. You have now completed this portion of the routine. Remember to maintain stomach contraction as often as comfortably possible.

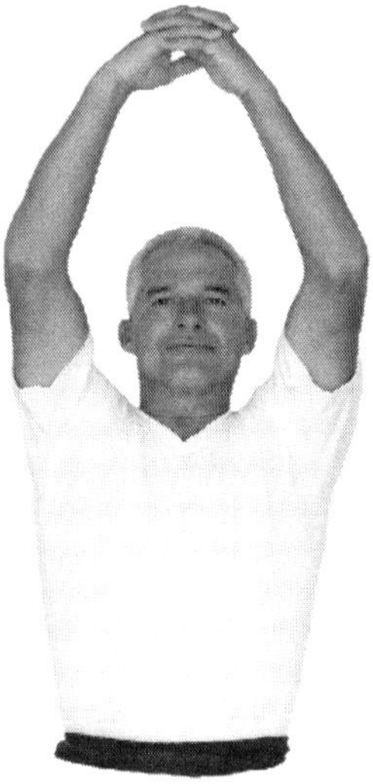
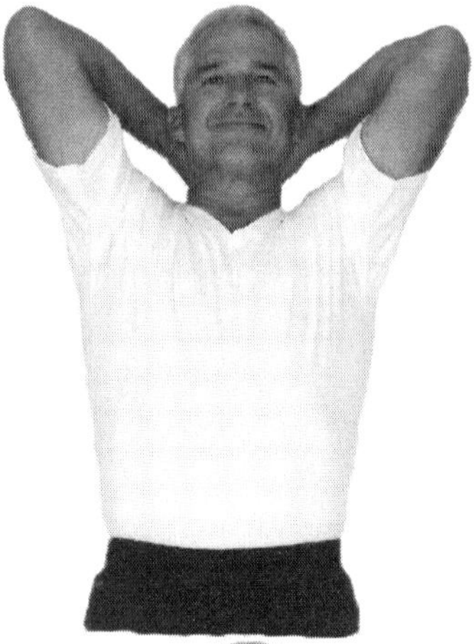
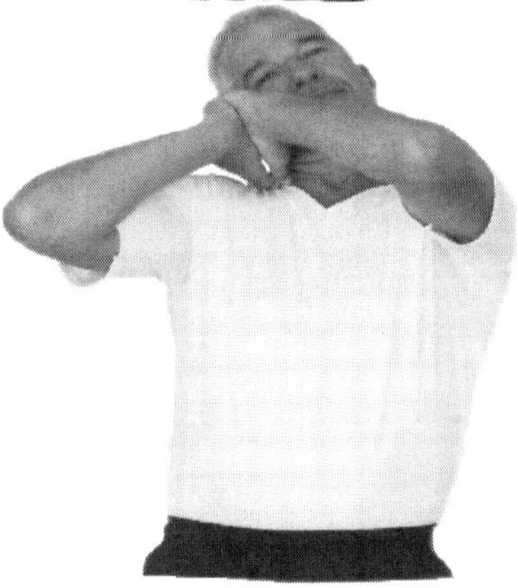
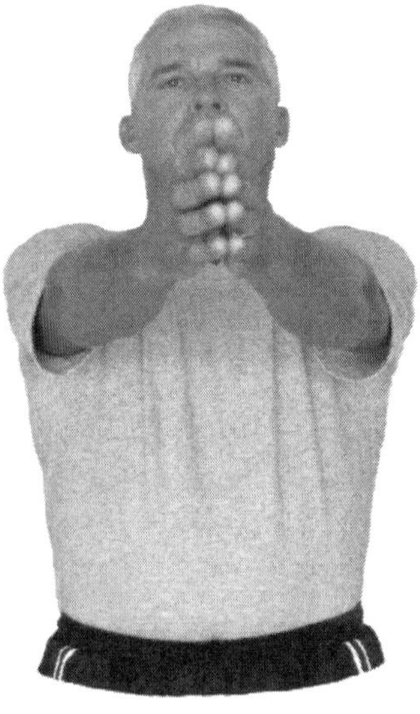
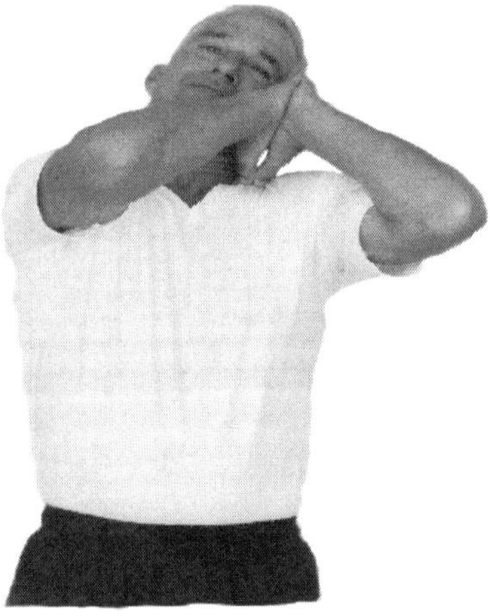

Upper Body

The following portion of the routine energizes muscles in the arms, across chest, and shoulders. Cross the fingers or attempt to touch, and raise the arms up over your head. Straighten them upward as much as possible. This is the starting position.

Bending the elbows, slowly lower the hands down and behind the head wrists kept straight, trying to touch the neck, pause. No need to force them to touch. Slowly raise the hands back overhead to the original starting position, for a count of one. Repeat movement a total of ten times.

This next segment will energize the neck and facial muscles. Maintain the previous contact with the hands. Lower the arms down from overhead until they are pointed straight out at the shoulders in front of the body. At this point uncross the fingers, extend them out straight and allow the palms of the hands and fingers to lie flat against each other. This is the starting position for this portion of the routine.

Bend both arms at the elbow up, raising the forearms up and back to the right side of the head. Place the back side of the left hand next to the right side of the neck, leaving a little space between the hands and neck. Slowly lean the head to the right until it touches the hands, pause. Slowly raise the head back upright using the neck muscles. Do not push the head back upright with the hands. Rotate the elbows forward returning the hands out in front to the starting position for a count of one. Repeat this movement to the opposite or left side of the neck, leaving a little space between the hands and neck. Slowly lean the head to the left until it touches the hands, pause. Slowly raise the head back upright using the neck muscles. Do not push the head back upright with the hands. Return hands to the starting position. Increment the count by one each time the hands return to their starting position. Repeat move to the opposite side each time for a total of ten, five times each side.

21

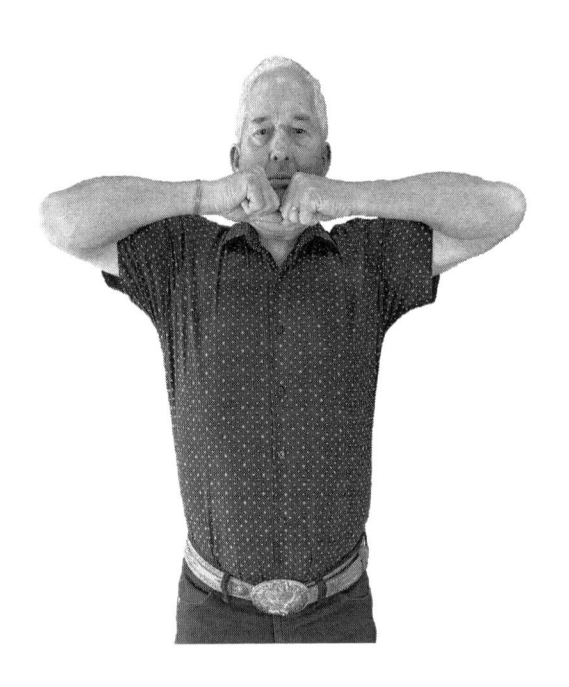

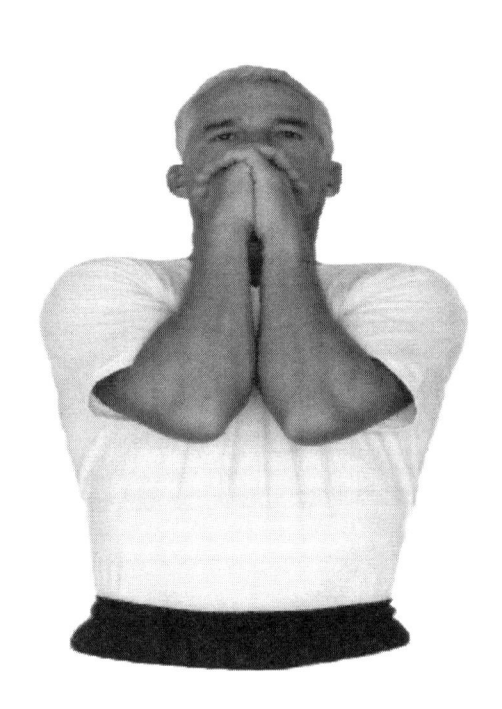

The final upper body routine works the chest muscles, shoulders, across the back, and both arms. From the starting position of the previous segment, bend the arms at the elbow, raising the hands up and back toward the face. At this time, change the contact of the hands back to the fingers being crossed. Bring the crossed fingers back to the face and place them partially under the chin.

With the chin resting upon the crossed fingers, raise the elbows out to the side of the body. The forearms should be parallel to the ground. This is the starting position.

Slowly lower the elbows, bringing the forearms together in front of the chest, pause. The attempting to touch will also work. Slowly move the elbows back out away from each other, returning to the starting position, for a count of one. Repeat movement a total of ten times.

For women, the lowering of the arms can be alternated a little higher or lower as needed per individual. The higher or lower motions will increase muscle toning across the upper and side supporting chest muscles as well as across the back.

The first things noticed as a result of doing the upper body portion of the routine is the reduction of tense, sore muscles associated with stress, improved range of motion and increased energy level. It is also removing excess facial fat providing one with a more youthful appearance. All this while slowly removing excess body fat.

23

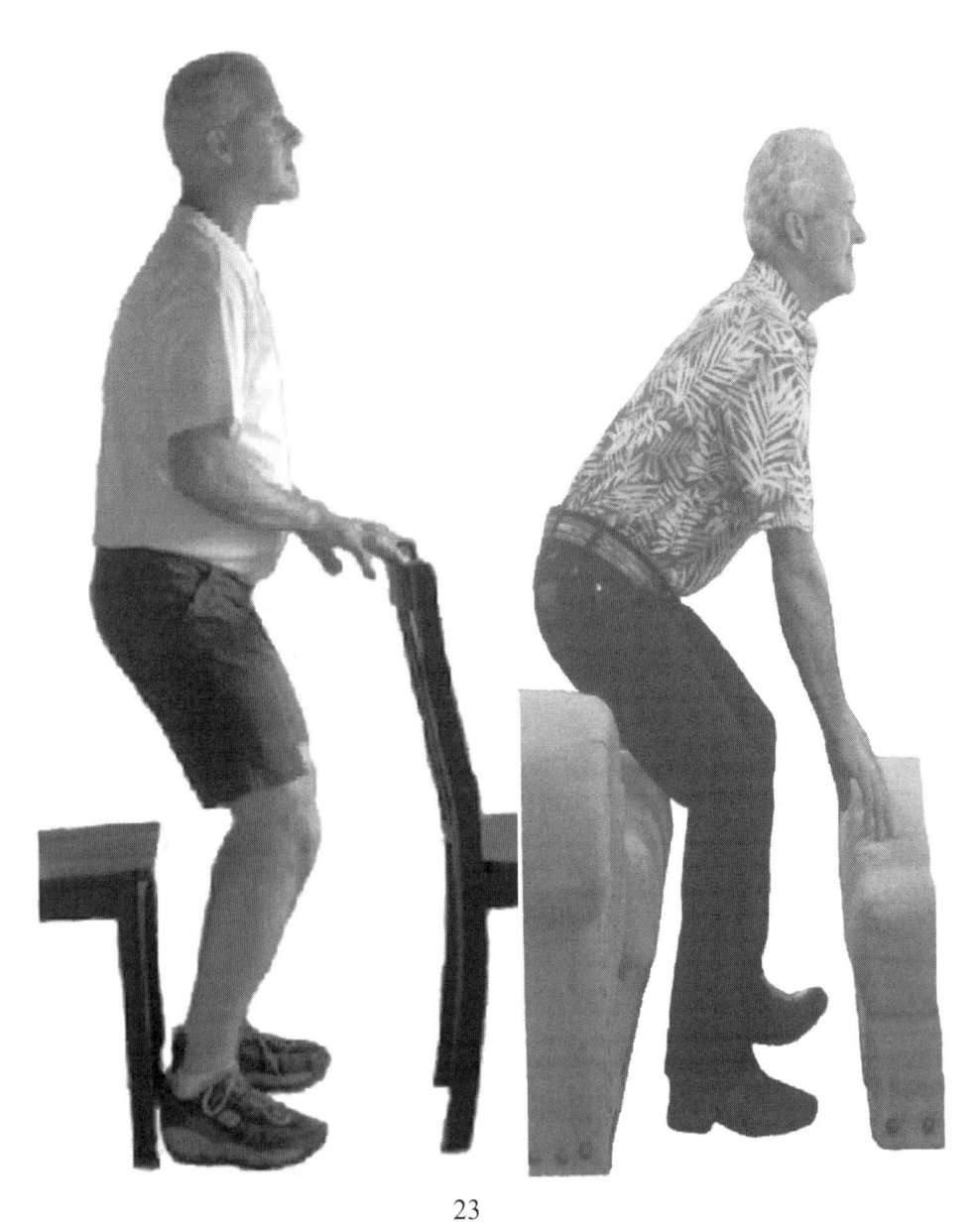

Lower Body

The lower body routine works muscles in the legs and buttocks while providing some cardiovascular workout. With the lower body portion of the routine, a stationary object is used to help position the weight of the upper body onto the buttocks and legs. Examples are the edge of a table, back or arm of a chair, anything around hip height. The routine is done in front of a chair or sofa to allow for sitting down if needed.

Stand facing the object chosen, allowing room for comfortable movement. From this location, bend the knees and lower the buttocks approximately three inches into a partially squatting stance. Extend both arms out and lightly touch the stationary surface. Position the upper body weight onto the legs and buttocks. The support and balance control of your weight is on the legs, not on the stationary surface. This is the starting position for the lower body movement.

From this slightly squatted position slowly squat the legs, lowering the buttocks and upper body three more inches pausing. Slowly raise, using the legs, back to the original starting position. This is for a count of one. Repeat the downward and upward moves until a total of fifteen is reached. If in the beginning the upper body weight is too much to do fifteen, do a lesser amount. Try to start with at least three if possible. Increase the number until fifteen is reached. This is a slow gliding motion using the legs and buttocks to support the weight of the upper body. This will also produce a slight increase in the rate of the heartbeat.

This slow-paced, continuous moving routine starts with the stomach, moves to the upper body, then down to the lower body to make one set. One set takes around three minutes. Repeat the routine two more times, completing the program in about ten minutes. Allow a little time between each set before repeating. Remember this can also be done while watching TV. When a commercial comes on, do a set. After three commercials the program is completed.

Made in the USA
Columbia, SC
12 October 2024